Thyroid Guide:

Thyroid Facts and Food Recommendations

By

Debra Helton

ISBN-13: 978-1495494437

Table of Contents

Introduction 5

Chapter 1. Where Is The Thyroid? 6

Chapter 2. Thyroid Facts 7

    Potential Causes Of Thyroid Disease 10

Chapter 3. Foods That Help A Slow Thyroid (Hypothyroidism) . 11

Chapter 4. Foods That Can Help A Fast Thyroid (Hyperthyroidism) 13

Chapter 5. Foods to Avoid 15

Chapter 6. Thyroid Diet Meal Plan 18

    1. Breakfast Diet Plan 19

    2. Lunch Diet Plan 21

    3. Dinner Diet Plan 25

    4. Snacks 28

Conclusion 31

Thank You Page 33

Thyroid Diet Guide: Thyroid Facts and Food Recommendations

By Debra Helton

© Copyright 2013 Debra Helton

Reproduction or translation of any part of this work beyond that permitted by section 107 or 108 of the 1976 United States Copyright Act without permission of the copyright owner is unlawful. Requests for permission or further information should be addressed to the author.

This publication is designed to provide accurate and authoritative information in regard to the subject matter covered. This work is sold with the understanding that the publisher is not engaged in rendering legal, accounting, or other professional services. If legal advice or other expert assistance is required, the services of a competent professional person should be sought.

First Published, 2013

Printed in the United States of America

Introduction

The thyroid is a gland in the body that stores hormones that help to regulate your heart rate, body temperature, blood pressure, and also the rate that at which your body will convert food into energy. Taking care of your thyroid is very important and so you need to understand that it does require maintenance and a lot of information. Having a good thyroid diet will ensure that you will be very healthy and your body is functioning correctly. Thyroid hormones are very important for every cell in your body and so it is crucial for children to grow up and for adults to stay healthy.

The book Thyroid Diet Guide: Thyroid Facts and Food Recommendations gives you actual information about thyroid as well as helps you to stay healthy.

Chapter 1. Where Is The Thyroid?

The thyroid is located towards the lower part of your neck and this is under the Adam's apple. It is in the shape of a butterfly and there are two lobes that are attached to the middle. The thyroid actually uses iodine and this is a mineral that is found in most foods and also in iodized salt. The important thyroid hormones would be thyroxine and also triiodothyronine. The thyroid stimulating hormones are produced by the pituitary gland and will help stimulate hormone production.

Chapter 2. Thyroid Facts

Many experts have recently estimated that over many 59 million Americans are currently suffering from thyroid conditions such as Hashimoto's Disease, thyroid nodules, Graves' disease, hyperthyroidism, hypothyroidism, and thyroid cancer. It is highly crucial for doctors and patients to broaden their knowledge about all these common and frequently overlooked hormonal health problems so that people can be able to prevent symptoms from worsening. According to many thyroid patient advocates and experts, many doctors simply do not communicate with patients about their potential thyroid risks, diagnosis, symptoms, and treatments.

It is very alarming on how millions of people currently are suffering from these thyroid conditions, but the worst part is that they're not getting any proper diagnosed treatment. Many have been wondering whether it is a lack of knowledge on the doctors part or the lack of interest patients have on actually getting treatment. Some have also stated that those suffering from these conditions lose interest in treating their thyroid problems because of the high costs for treatment.

To help overcome the lack of information and knowledge on the topic, it is important for everyone who can attain any thyroid problems to eat healthier. By knowing what foods can keep your thyroid healthy, you may likely help prevent the symptoms from worsening.

Your thyroid is a tiny butterfly-shaped gland that has an enormous responsibility when it comes with your body's natural metabolic function. Specifically, your thyroid needs to release two primary hormones which are triiodothyronine and thyroxine. These two hormone are in control with your metabolism so if anything goes wrong, it can havoc your metabolism's entire movement.

When the metabolism is working properly, then these hormones will travel throughout your bloodstream to help the cells get the needed amount of energy from the foods that you eat. Your thyroid hormones are responsible for the natural regulating of your blood calcium levels and body temperature. These hormones are needed to help with the development and growth of proper brain development.

For many Americans, the thyroid produces are either too little or too much hormones, which then causes a dozen health symptoms that can get severe. However, because thyroid diseases are often misdiagnosed or are even overlooked, it is estimated that over half of Americans that are affected by the disease have no idea their thyroid is suffering medically.

Women are considered to be more prone to getting thyroid problems compared to males, where around one out of five women develop thyroid problems in their lifetime. The risk of this condition increases as you age while genetics also plays a huge role when it comes to attaining the condition.

Potential Causes Of Thyroid Disease

1. Having autoimmune disease or being near relative with the condition
2. Radiation exposure
3. Going through pre-menopause or menopause
4. Thyroid surgery
5. Recently giving birth

Chapter 3. Foods That Help A Slow Thyroid (Hypothyroidism)

1. Sea Weed

Seaweed is naturally rich with iodine and also other trace minerals that can help speed up a slow thyroid. This has been a very popular food among those that want to have a healthier thyroid and so it certainly has been proven to help. In the past, native people would go through a lot of trouble to try and obtain seaweed from the sea and this would help them avoid goiter. Since iodine is very important for thyroid functions and health, it is very helpful to have seaweed in your diet.

If you do not have the right amount of iodine, then your body will not be able to create the needed the thyroid hormones. It is equally important to understand that too much of anything can be dangerous and so you need to keep this in mind. Moderation is important for any diet and it is just as crucial for a healthy thyroid diet.

2. Coconut Oil

Coconut oil has been able to help support thyroid function because it will slightly stimulate the production of thyroid hormones in your body and in your metabolism. Adding coconut oil into your diet will help you to support your thyroid health and also be very beneficial for those that suffer from hypothyroidism to also lose weight. This food also helps to reduce cholesterol for those that have hypothyroidism. Since saturated fat helps promote thyroid function, coconut oil does its job because it is largely comprised of just that.

3. Shellfish

Just like most vegetables, shellfish is very rich in iodine and so it is very helpful for thyroid production. If you were to add a food that tastes good and has a good amount of iodine, this just might be the best option.

Chapter 4. Foods That Can Help A Fast Thyroid (Hyperthyroidism)

1. Fermented Soy Foods

Most people will admit that soy is a very healthy food and it's not a surprise that it can also help with those that may have thyroid problems. Soy is goitrogenic and it is a very strong suppressor of your thyroid hormones. There has been research that indicates that soy can be more effective than most anti-thyroid drugs and so this may be surprising for most people. Soy is also a very potent food and so this means that it is very strong and so it can help those in need.

2. Raw Vegetables

It is obvious that vegetables are indeed healthy but it seems like people are just not able to understand that it is also very helpful for those that may have thyroid problems. A thyroid diet is just not complete without raw cruciferous vegetables and so you need to consider adding this to your diet if you are serious about being able to help your thyroid stay healthy.

There are plenty of vegetables to choose from but cabbage, turnips, and brussels are only some of the many that you need to consider. These vegetables have goitrogens and so this will interfere with the iodine uptake and this will then interfere with your thyroid producing hormones

3. Millet

Just like vegetables, Millets are very nutritious but they also have a lot goitrogens that will help interfere your thyroid's iodine uptake. This is very helpful and when you cook millets, it will also help mitigate the anti thyroid effects a bit.

Chapter 5. Foods to Avoid

When it comes to creating the perfect thyroid diet, you need to keep in mind that you need to know whether or not you have a slow or fast thyroid. However, no matter what kind of thyroid you have, it is important to skip on these foods.

1. Gluten-containing grains
Recent studies have been able to show that there is a very obvious connection between thyroid disease and celiac disease and so this greatly proves the point that gluten-containing grains are not for those that want to eat healthy for their diet. Those that suffer from autoimmune thyroid disease will have a higher chance of suffering from celiac disease and so this is quite scary.

What's fascinating though is that a diet that will not have any gluten can make anti-thyroid antibodies disappear in just 3-6 months. This is incredible because this is a natural way to getting rid of those annoying anti-bodies. This means that you really need to consider removing wheat, barley, and several other grains that may contain gluten from your diet if you happen to suffer from autoimmune thyroid disease.

2. Unfermented Soy

Though soy is generally healthy, unfermented soy is not. Unfermented soy that is rich in concentrated genistein and isoflavones will actually contribute to you getting autoimmune thyroid disease. With unfermented soy, it can do a lot of damage to the thyroid. If you need to eat soy, make sure you are eating it in small portions and keep in mind that the fermented form is a lot better. Too much soy can be very bad for anyone and particularly someone with a thyroid problem.

3. Coffee

Coffee may seem like a harmless drink but it is not the best for those that suffer from either hyper or hypothyroidism. Since coffee is a very strong stimulant, it can really cause problems for those that are having trouble with hyperthyroidism because that's the last thing that they need. Coffee can also interfere with iodine uptake and this can stop the production of thyroid hormones and this can be a big problem. This is bad news for everyone that wants to keep their thyroid healthy.

4. Balance Is Always The Key

Just like with everything else, the key is to always focus balance and making sure you are not eating too much of the same foods or ignoring one food that you might need. Most people make the horrible mistake of trying to try a certain diet that they have never heard of and then hope that it will help them. It takes a lot of patience to learn all of these things but it is possible in the end.

Chapter 6. Thyroid Diet Meal Plan

Foods included in a thyroid diet meal plan

A thyroid diet meal plan is a meal plan for the foods that a person with underactive thyroid may eat. It consists of foods rich in iodine since iodine is known to curb the symptoms of hypothyroidism. Iodine is found in foods that we usually eat and are easy to find in most grocery stores and markets. The foods included in the list are seaweeds, seafood, iodized salt, saltwater fish, Celtic sea salt and sushi. And along with iodine, deficiency in the element selenium is also seen in patients with hypothyroidism. Therefore eating selenium-rich foods may also help like meat, chicken, tuna, salmon, whole unrefined grains, dairy products, onions and garlic.

1. Breakfast Diet Plan

Breakfast is the most important meal of the day and foods that are rich in iodine and selenium may be already be served.

Sample breakfast plan 1 – tuna in oil on whole wheat bread, a glass of milk and a slice of melon. 3 ounces of tuna in oil or about half a can of tuna contains 17mcg of iodine while wheat bread is a food rich in selenium. Melon slices contain vitamins.

Plan 2 – egg salad in whole wheat bread, a cup of fruit salad, a glass of milk. 1 large hard-boiled egg has 12mcg of iodine, a cup of cow's milk contains 56mcg of iodine while a cup of fruit salad is a perfect way to take in vitamins and minerals.

Plan 3 – chicken sandwich, yoghurt and a cup of chopped apples. Chicken breast is a good source of selenium and niacin while yoghurt is rich in iodine. Chopped apples contain amazing amounts of polyphenols that also supports thyroid function.

Plan 4 – egg omelette with onions, parsley and red bell peppers, a cup of cow's milk and a cup of Brazil nuts. Egg contains about 12mcg of iodine while onions and parsley contain polyphenol and red bell peppers contain vitamin C to boost the function of the thyroid gland. A cup of cow's milk contain about 56mcg of iodine and Brazil nuts are a rich source of selenium

Plan 5 – Cod in mayonnaise on a toasted whole wheat bread, a ripe banana and a cup of milk. About 3 ounces of cod contain 99mcg of iodine while whole wheat bread is a great source of selenium. A cup of cow's milk contains 56mcg of iodine and a banana is rich in vitamin B6 which is needed for normal function of the thyroid glands.

2. Lunch Diet Plan

Lunch time meal plans for patients diagnosed with hypothyroidism are delicious, colourful and varied. Since most nutritious and tasty meats contain significant amounts of selenium and iodine you will certainly enjoy eating. There are no drastic changes to your normal or traditional diet when you use the following lunch time meal plans:

Sample meal plan 1 – Brown rice with avocado slices and tomatoes, tuna slices in oil and green tea. Brown rice contains and avocadoes contain excellent amounts of vitamin B6 needed for normal thyroid function while canned tuna in oil will give you 17mcg of iodine. Green tea is rich in polyphenols also needed for improving thyroid function.

To cook brown rice, follow package instructions; mixed cooked rice with cherry tomatoes, avocadoes, minced cloves of garlic, freshly squeezed lemon juice and drizzle with extra virgin olive oil which is also rich in polyphenols.

Plan 2 – sautéed shrimps in butter and garlic, brown rice and a small bowl of fruit salad with cream. About 3 ounce of shrimp contains 35mcg of iodine while brown rice has niacin and vitamin B6 needed for optimum thyroid function. Fruits like kiwi, mangoes, oranges, cantaloupes and cherries contain significant amounts of polyphenols and vitamin B6.

Wash 2 ounces of shrimp and then remove the shell. Heat a sautéing pan and place the butter in the pan and then sauté shrimps. Brown rice should be cooked according to its instructions on the packaging.

Plan 3 – fried chicken, mashed potatoes and a slice of cantaloupe. Chicken contains great amounts of Selenium while potatoes are rich in vitamin B6. Cantaloupes are not just sweet and tasty but are also rich in polyphenols and vitamin c to improve thyroid function.

Marinate chicken in lemon juice, freshly ground pepper, salt and crushed garlic. Allow to marinate in about 12 hours. When chicken is ready, dip in egg and roll in flour for crispy fried chicken. Boil 2 to 3 large potatoes in a huge pot of water; when potatoes are ready mash them with a masher. Then place these in a large bowl and combine with a cup of milk, freshly ground pepper and salt.

Plan 4 – sautéed salmon with tomatoes, pineapples and onions, brown rice and a cup of frozen berries. Salmon is one of the richest sources of iodine while brown rice is a perfect source of vitamin B6 and polyphenols needed for normal thyroid development. Onions and tomatoes also contain polyphenols and vitamin C respectively and are needed for boosting the function of the thyroid glands. Frozen berries are rich sources of vitamins and minerals needed for improving thyroid health.

Chop onions and tomatoes; use about 3 ounces of salmon about the size of a pack of cards. Drain a can of pineapple chunks. Saute all the ingredients and then add salmon pieces. Add a dash of pepper and salt. Cook brown rice as per package instructions. Freeze berries overnight and then add cream when you are ready to eat.

Plan 5 – sushi rolls, ripe mangoes and iced tea. Sushi is known to have tremendous amounts of iodine specifically the seaweed wrap which has 4.5mcg of iodine per ¼ ounce. Sushi rolls contain different types of fish and seafood but you may also make your own sushi roll at home. Use a sushi mat, a large seaweed wrap, sushi rice, and your choice of deep sea fish ingredients. First place the mat on a flat surface, place the seaweed wrap and then scatter the newly cooked rice over the wrap. Make sure that rice is perfectly arranged and then add your choice of ingredients. Roll the sushi tightly and then slice it into bite sized pieces. Ripe mangoes may be sliced in thirds with the two fleshy portions sliced vertically and horizontally. Serve this dish as soon as you are done.

3. Dinner Diet Plan

Dinner is a time to relax and enjoy meals with the family. You can use these thyroid meal plans for dinner every day of the week:

Sample meal plan 1 – roasted salmon, eggplant with guacamole dip and fruit salad medley. Salmon is rich in iodine, eggplants are high in polyphenols, guacamole is made of avocadoes, tomatoes and onions which are all foods that will benefit people with thyroid conditions.

A classic guacamole recipe is made of 2 avocadoes, a tomato, a small onion, a clove of garlic, a dash of fresh lemon juice, small pieces of cilantro and salt to taste. Chop all the ingredients into very small pieces and then place all the ingredients in a bowl; top this with cilantro leaves.

Plan 2 – steamed snapper, steamed vegetables, a bowl of frozen berries. Snappers are high in selenium while veggies (except for broccoli and cabbages) are rich in nutrients needed for a healthy thyroid.

Rub salt and pepper on either side of the snapper and steam to perfection. Steam the veggies together with the snapper in a portable steamer. Add a piece of butter over the snapper and the veggies for more flavour. Freeze the berries in the fridge the night before and serve chilled.

Plan 3 – vegetable soup, goat cheese salad, iced tea and fruits in season. This vegetable soup has ingredients that contain vitamins and minerals for better thyroid function. Goat cheese salad is a perfect source of the amino acid Tyrosine which is very important for a healthy thyroid.

Vegetable soup is made of a finely chopped medium onion, grated large carrot, 1 finely chopped leek, 4 grated small potatoes, vegetable stock, a can of Flageolet beans, salt and pepper and extra virgin olive oil. Sauté the onion in extra virgin olive oil and then add the carrots and potatoes and cook for 5 minutes. Afterwards add the leek, celery and the vegetable stock cube. When this boils, place in a blender and blend to the desired consistency. Place the mixture in a pot and continue cooking, add the beans and then cook for another 2 minutes. Remove from heat and cook before serving.

Plan 4 – tuna fish sticks dipped in lima bean humus, apples and ice tea. 2 tuna fish sticks contain 35mcg while lima beans also contain high amounts of iodine. Apples are a great source of polyphenols which are also essential in thyroid function.

Tuna fish sticks are available in your local supermarket. Lima beans humus is made of a can of lima beans, about 1/3 fresh lemon juice, 2 cloves of minced garlic, a/2 teaspoon of cumin (ground), 1/3 cup of finely chopped parsley, salt and a tablespoon of paprika powder.

Blend all the ingredients together in a blender with medium speed except for parsley. After the mixture has the consistency that you desire then it is time to add the parsley and then blend in medium speed again.

Plan 5 – deep fried shrimp, steamed vegetables and berry shake. About 3 ounces of shrimps contain 35mcg of iodine while steamed veggies contain minerals and vitamins that can improve overall health and increase the function of underactive thyroids. Berries contain vitamin C that will also benefit the thyroid.

4. Snacks

For snacks, there are delicious and nutritious food alternatives that can make your thyroid healthier.

a) Hard boiled eggs are perfect for salads, sandwiches or you may eat it on its own. A large egg contains about 12mcg of iodine. Eggs also contain high amounts of protein that is needed for tissue repair, building muscles and better nerve function. Hard boiled eggs are also easy to cook and are easiest to take anywhere. You may also use any kind of condiments to eat hard boiled eggs like mayonnaise, ketchup, salt or pepper.

b) Brazil nuts are crunchy and nutritious since it contains selenium. You can make brownies, cookies, pesto and cake out of these nuts. You can also take Brazil nuts anywhere you go. Simply place it in a resealable plastic bag or a covered container and much on these for snacks.

c) Apples contain polyphenols that will also enhance thyroid function. You may eat apple from the tree or you may chop it and blend it to make apple sauce. Slice apples into thin slices to make apple pie. You can also press apples to yield apple juice.

d) Cherries, blackberries and blueberries are also rich sources of polyphenols. You can eat berries on their own or you may also use them as pie filling, for spreads, as preserves or to make smoothies. You may also combine berries and freeze them in small cups. Serve chilled topped with cream.

e) Sunflower seeds contain selenium and vitamin B6 that also strengthens thyroid function. You may eat roasted sunflower seeds for snacks or you may try adding these to your green salad, in baking breads, in sautéed vegetable and in cookies.

f) Oranges are rich in vitamin C that also boosts thyroid function thereby curbing symptoms of hypothyroidism. Oranges may be eaten on its own, sliced and added to different dishes, squeezed to make orange juice, ice pops and so much more. You may also try eating mandarins and tangerines.

g) Peanuts are rich in vitamin E that combines with zinc and vitamin A to be able to produce thyroid hormones.

You may eat peanuts after it has been cooked. You may add peanuts to different dishes, pastries, cakes, cookies and so many more. You may grind fresh peanuts into peanut butter or make peanut candy.

h) Sweet potatoes contain vitamin B6 that will help improve thyroid function. You can make fries out of sweet potatoes as well as sweet potato hash, pancakes and dips.

Conclusion

Now you know the basics of creating a good thyroid diet but the last thing is to put all of this together. You need to take some time every week to gather the right foods and then see if you have everything there. The next thing is to then start adding these foods to your diet so that you are seemingly adding healthier foods to your diet without completely changing everything. This is very helpful because you will see that it is not that simple. You will be adding healthy foods for your diet without having to feel like you are making a life change. When you are able to have all the foods, the last thing is to then start coming up with recipes.

The internet is full of recipes that you can make and some of them will actually target your certain thyroid problem. With the internet's information, it is nearly impossible to not find the best recipes out there because it is definitely worth it. Most people will try to just workout or eat less food to become healthy but this is not the way. The goal is to simply add new foods and then see if it will make a difference. This is a very easy and effective way to help keep your thyroid healthy at all times.

Before you make any big changes in your life, you must consult your doctor. None of this information should override what your doctor has given you as this is simply a guideline for those that want a place to start. Though the information is indeed legitimate and you will find that everything is correct, it is still very important that you talk to your doctor or nutritionist. When you do talk to them, let them know about the information that you learned and then ask them if they fully agree. Have a long talk with your doctor and then you will learn how to make the best possible thyroid diet for your certain condition.

Thank You Page

I want to personally thank you for reading my book. I hope you found information in this book useful and I would be very grateful if you could leave your honest review about this book. I certainly want to thank you in advance for doing this.

Printed in Great Britain
by Amazon.co.uk, Ltd.,
Marston Gate.